French Secrets about Diet, Fitness & Wellness

"Like The French" *Series, Book 1*

Lesleigh Kivedo

French Secrets about Diet, Fitness & Wellness

Copyright © 2018

ISBN: 9781977036612

Warning and Disclaimer

Publisher Contact

Skinny Bottle Publishing
books@skinnybottle.com

SKINNY
BOTTLE

Lesleigh Kivedo:

A self-confessed Francophile at heart, Lesleigh Kivedo has been writing about fashion, beauty, health and travel for over 10 years. Starting her career as an editorial intern at *Marie Claire* magazine (yes, like Anne Hathaway in *The Devil Wears Prada*), she then found her fashion feet as a features writer for *Cosmopolitan* magazine in South Africa. Her travels have since taken her to Montreal, Amsterdam, Bali, Dubai and, of course, her beloved Paris. These days, when not re-watching *Paris Je T'aime*, she continues with her passion for writing as a lifestyle journalist, covering everything from the up-and-coming fashion tendencies to the latest Kimye baby.

French Food, Fitness & Wellness

Introduction

Just by looking at French women, you might think they all share the same magical skinny gene. How else can they live among all that cheese, wine and baguettes and still look like waifish gamines?

It's been labeled the French Paradox – the fact that the average French person's daily diet is laden with cheese, butter, bread and wine, yet they have the lowest rate of obesity in the world. Even more surprising: they live longer and suffer from fewer coronary heart diseases than any other country, regardless of consuming copious levels of full-fat dairy products, butter-drenched breads, and cholesterol-heavy meats.

First things first though – this is not a diet book. If anything, it's a moderation book. That is, you can eat whatever you like as long as it's in moderation. There is a principle in business known as the 80/20 rule. The French diet can be regarded in pretty much the same way: eat healthily 80 percent of the time and the remaining 20 percent lets you treat yourself with your favorite "cheat" foods. Simply put, focus on eating three balanced, nutritious meals every day and you're free to splurge on those beloved chocolate bars and glasses of red wine. "You can't be 100 percent all of the time, but you can be 80 percent all of the time," so says Yumi Lee, a Los Angeles-based personal trainer credited with helping celebrities like Jessica Alba and Miranda Kerr stay in shape.

Moderation, that's what it all boils down to... and a talent for keeping their stay-slim tricks to themselves. According to beauty and style guru Caroline de Maigret, there is one thing that all French women have in common - they know how to keep a secret. "It's funny because we don't talk about those things—you don't say you're on a diet or that you go to the gym," she told *Vogue*. "And you don't look like you have a lot of makeup on, even if it took

you a good half-hour to do it. It's all in moderation."

In her co-authored book *How to Be Parisian Wherever You Are: Love, Style, and Bad Habits,* de Maigret goes on to explain the difference in the way that the French see life as a whole. "I think it's just part of our culture—we're used to not having a Prince Charming. You see how people act in life and we don't lie to ourselves...It's OK to have wrinkles, but we treat ourselves so that we look better... We realize that there is no ideal and that chasing an ideal is exhausting."

So, what's the answer? Enjoy the face, the body, the life that you have. "I think what's sort of shifting [on the beauty landscape] is 'beauty from within,'" said fashion buyer Marlo Sutton, speaking to *Into the Gloss*. Although Canadian by birth, she can now rightfully be considered an honorary Parisian, having lived in the city for 13 years. "A really healthy diet, drinking a lot of water, taking supplements, exercise – that's the starting point to having a freshness and a glow."

With this in mind, we've compiled a go-to guide on all things diet, fitness, and wellness related - with a French spin. *Bon Appétit!*

FOOD

Remember the book *French Women Don't Get Fat?* The 2004 bestseller may have been only 304 pages long, but it may as well have been a movement.

It sparked a revolution. Suddenly a spotlight was shone on these much-admired albeit oft misunderstood lifestyle ingénues. All their dietary hacks, fitness manifestos, and wellbeing mantras were revealed in one tell-all tome.

Author Mireille Guiliano received a fair deal of backlash for her no-nonsense views. "The real reason French women don't get fat is not genetic, but cultural," she said. "And if the French subjected themselves to the American extremes of eating and dieting, the obesity problem in France would be much worse than what has struck America." Harsh? Maybe. But consider the merits of the French lifestyle she promotes. "French women typically think about good things to eat. American women typically worry about bad things to eat."

So, does it all come down to mindset? It would appear so, along with a few definitive lifestyle changes - all of which begin with that distinctly French philosophy: balance.

Tout est question d'équilibre

(It's all a question of balance)

French dining is not about deprivation – quite the opposite. "You can eat any good food in moderation . . . in three bites," so says Mireille Guilliano. All types of food are allowed in small doses. "It's okay to have a glass of wine, good bread, or a few bites of dessert. It's about how you pick your moment."

The common denominator among French dining is an appreciation for the food that they eat. Instead of large quantities at mealtimes, there is a focus on the quality instead. Take eating in a restaurant, for example. You'd be hard-pressed to find words like "bottomless" or "all-you-can-eat" on a standard French menu. That is simply not *de rigueur.*

No, the portion sizes in France are considerably smaller than in other countries. One reason for this may be an old French custom that says it's extremely bad manners to leave food on your dinner plate. This is seen as insulting to the chef and has resulted in many French eateries now offering take-away or "le doggy bag" to their clients (although still regarded with a sneer as an American vulgarity).

Something else that might seem a foreign concept, especially when regarding their casual approach to looking good? "French women don't get fat because they are obsessed with weight." So says tell-it-like-is beauty publicist Marie-Laure Fournier. Speaking to *The Cut*, she explained her experience with American beauty editors. "It's funny because I was with a girlfriend and I was like... I eat less than you, and you are smaller than me!' But the trick is that if she or a French woman goes out for dinner, she will eat soup for lunch. One of the meals is extremely light. I was in Paris in April and already the magazines had stories about how to lose extra pounds for the summer."

Take Audrey Hepburn as an example. She may not have been born French, but given her fondness for the City of Lights, we'd like to think of her as the artist's imagination of the typical Parisienne. According to her son Luca Dotti: "She loved Italian food and pasta. She ate a lot of grains, not a lot of meat, and a little bit of everything," he told *People* magazine. "She had a healthy metabolism, but she was not excessive," added her longtime beau Robert Wolders. "She had chocolate after dinner, baking chocolate [and] she had a finger or two of Scotch at night."

The theme of moderation is one that has permeated through the years, with modern-day French women still adopting those same moderate sensibilities.

"I don't eat a lot of meat, but more because I don't really like it than anything else," actress Clémence Poésy told *British Vogue*. "I have friends who are vegans for their own reasons and I think that as long as food remains a pleasure then you can do whatever you want to do. I'm not a fan of rules as such - I think people should be able to do what they want. My dad's family had a farm which my uncle took over and turned into an organic farm. So, I try to eat what's in season and try to buy products that are natural, and that are produced fairly. And I'm aware of what a luxury it is to be able to do that, and to make those decisions."

Renowned French style writer Garance Doré is based in New York but still remembers her French upbringing. "I come from the South and the famous Mediterranean diet (vegetables, fish, rice, olive oil) makes me very happy! I've tried to adapt it to my life in New York, but it isn't easy," she told *Vogue Paris*.

"I am from the coast, so I love fish, seafood etcetera," quips Elite Model Look winner (and face of Chanel Chance) Charlotte di Calypso, speaking to *WomenFitness.net*. "But I also love bread and cheese (as a good "frenchie"). So, my advice is to eat a little bit of everything to keep your body and your mind happy!"

If all else fails, remember the words of iconic supermodel Linda Evangelista. She might not be a native Parisienne but as the one-time muse of Chanel's Karl Lagerfeld, she has the lifestyle down pat. Her diet mantra? "I don't diet. I just don't eat as much as I'd like to."

GROCERY SHOPPING LIKE A FRENCHIE

It's no secret that portion sizes in the US are somewhat larger than in the rest of the world. Did you know, however, that refrigerators are bigger too? Or rather... let's rephrase that. The refrigerators in France are considerably smaller than those in the US and many other parts of the world. Why? There is simply no need to have a big one when all you do is fill it up on a meal-to-meal basis.

The food stored in the fridge is of the perishable variety and will be consumed within one or two days in any case. Every day involves a visit to *le marché* or market - usually specialty stalls that focus on one area of fresh produce: the bakery or *la boulangerie*, the butchery or *le bucherie*, la fromagerie (cheese shop) ... you get the idea. Of course, there are supermarkets too like Monoprix and Carrefour but even these focus on high-quality items. Don't be surprised if you don't find a wide selection of products to choose from either. Unlike elsewhere, the options are limited and for good reason.

American food author Michael Ruhlman described the phenomena he has witnessed in US grocery stores in his book *Grocery: The Buying and Selling of Food in America*. He outlines the wide range of packaged, processed foods he has witnessed on US shelves - all 40 000 of them. "In the past couple of decades, it's gone up from about 7,000. Food manufacturers have found that they can increase demand and sell more products if they give you more variety," he says. "It represents the extraordinary luxury that Americans have at our fingertips, seven days a week."

The situation in France could not be more different. The average French shopper knows what she came to the store to buy: ingredients for her next meal. She will rarely be swayed by gimmicks or promotional deals. If she doesn't need it that day, she won't buy it.

It might even be a clever trick in keeping the weight off. If your fridge and cupboards are bare of snacks and ready-to-eat meals, you'll have less temptation to give in to convenience. Your only options will be either to eat that leftover leek soup or make a special trip to the store. Then we haven't even mentioned the amount of money you will find yourself saving - all the more to spend on those expensive gourmet treats you just can't live without.

CHOOSE FRESH FOOD (UNLESS IT'S AGED WINE OR FERMENTED CHEESE, THAT IS)

If there is one thing that the French know how to do very well, it's indulge and not feel guilty about it. Why? Well, why *not*? There is even a popular French proverb that goes: *Un jour sans vin est comme un jour sans soleil.* Translated into English, it says: A day without wine is like a day without sunshine. How quintessentially *français, non*?

The thinking goes, if you're going to eat, you might as well enjoy it, right? "I'm French. I love wine and cheese," says French model Cindy Bruna, speaking to Coveteur website. "I love cooking... I try to cook for myself almost every day when I'm home in Paris. But if I go to a restaurant, I'm going to splurge. I don't go out to order salad!"

Find those foods that make your body feel its best. Very soon, you'll learn what makes you feel sluggish, tired and generally *crevé*. "I try as much as possible to eat clean,"

French model Camille Hurel told *Vogue* magazine. "Our skin reflects what we eat and our habits—you can't lie with it!"

French model Sigrid Agren has a similar view. Speaking to *Vogue*, she explained: "I don't follow any particular diet, but of course I try to be healthy and I am conscious about buying products that are in-season, organic and local. I try to avoid processed foods. I eat a lot of vegetables, fruits, nuts, and whole grains. I also love fish after growing up Martinique and eating fresh fish almost every day. Most of all, I'd say I'm addicted to dark chocolate!"

This appreciation of natural ingredients carries across all ages, with even young adults choosing to prepare their own meals at home. A survey by the Committee for Health Education (CFES), a sector of the French government, found that 76% of people prepared most of their meals at home, with 75% of them choosing to sit around the table. Food, in general, is closely tied to the country's long-standing heritage of savoring good food and wine for pleasure and not necessity. The length of a meal averages around two hours long.

"For France, a meal is a very particular moment, in which you share pleasure, the food as well as the conversation,' according to Dr. Francoise L'Hermite, a nutritionist from Paris. "From an Anglo-Saxon point of view, food is just fuel to give energy to your muscles. If you have no pleasure in it, you are breaking all the rules of eating."

On the same token though, there is one area that French people will not skimp on: their wine. When asked about her ultimate comfort food, French jewelry designer Marie Poniatowski told *Vogue Paris*: "A glass of good Bordeaux (especially a Carbonnieux 2006)." Caudalie founder Mathilde Thomas lives along the same lines. Her diet regime? "A glass of red Smith Haut Lafitte wine every night!" she told *Vogue Paris*. "When possible, I try to cut down on sugar and eat salmon, broccoli, apples, and oatmeal." Then there is interior designer Sarah Lavoine who, when asked what she never goes to bed without, told the magazine: "With a glass of very good red!"

DETOX DOES THE BODY GOOD

Sonia Sieff is the daughter of iconic photographer Jeanloup Sieff. Herself an up-and-coming shutterbug, her daily life in the bohemian Montmartre district channels that laissez-faire *joie de vivre* we have come to associate with the modern French woman. Speaking to *Vogue Paris*, she heralded the wonders of water and the occasional fast. "Warm water and lemon juice on waking is a classic, otherwise, I like the idea of fasting. I must be good to give the body a break and the same goes for alcohol - the older I get the less I drink, it just wears you out."

Another cheerleader of the all-body detox is former French supermodel Estelle Lefébure. At the impressive age of 50, the once *Vogue* and *Elle* cover girl could give women half her age a run for their money. The name still not ring a bell? Look up George Michael's *Too Funky* music video. She's the edgy blonde femme fatale in skintight patent leather!

With years of lived-through experience, the statuesque blonde has put her thoughts to paper and penned a healthy lifestyle manual called *Mindful Beauty: How to Look and Feel Great in Every Season*.

What's her expert advice for getting your body (
sluggish rut? A 20-day organic lemon cure. It wo
this: bring two cups of water to the boil, adding one lemon
which has been sliced in two. Squeeze out the lemon into
the boiled water before straining it. Sip on this mixture all
throughout the day. Then comes day two. Follow the same
procedure, except this time, increase the dosage to two
lemons in the same quantity of water. Day three equals
three lemons and so forth until you reach day ten. On this
day, up the amount of water to six cups with ten lemons.

At this point, the dosage begins to decrease. On day
eleven, use nine lemons followed by eight lemons on day
twelve. Carry on cutting down the quantities until you
reach day twenty. This course does wonders to clear out
your liver and actively burn fat in the body. A bonus?
Radiantly glowing skin! Just ask the ever-beautiful French
actress Catherine Deneuve. "Every morning I drink lemon
juice," she told *Into the Gloss*. "It's not so much that it
cleanses anything, but I do think it's very good for your
skin and the whites of your eyes."

Other tips from Lefébure: cut down on your dairy intake
but do take a nutritional supplement of Milk Thistle. She
also administers dandelion greens and artichokes as
regular parts of her own diet - the former is an excellent
source of vitamin A while the latter helps to lower
cholesterol.

Her other natural superfood? Quince. "This fruit has many
antioxidant properties. Low in sugar and calories, it's also
a good source of copper and nutritional fiber. It can be
substituted for apricots in tagine recipes or you can
combine it with chestnuts or apples in compotes," she

says. Almonds too are a regular find in the supermodel's handbag. "They can be eaten as a healthy, high-protein snack. I like to eat them with fruit, but I avoid mixing them with starchy products such as cereal or cookies since I find it causes indigestion."

WATER AS A WAY OF LIFE

Good old H20. Meet any French woman on the street and you'll most likely find her armed and ready with a large bottle of water.

Unfortunately, it's one of those necessities that we only really pay attention to once it's lacking. Fashion buyer Marlo Sutton explained her newfound appreciation for water to *Into the Gloss*. "I just did this big trip in Peru and because of the altitude, I had to drink tons of water. I was drinking 4, 5 liters of water a day. It's amazing how much of a difference it made."

But it's not only water that keeps them going. Anything herbal, organic and busting with natural ingredients are preferable to processed drinks. "I drink genmaicha, a Japanese green tea made with puffed rice, all day," says interior design Sarah Lavoine. Weird? Maybe. Healthy? Most definitely.

"I drink liters and liters of herbal tea and water," renowned Parisian fashion blogger Jeanne Damas told *Vogue*. And when you invariably imbibe, remember to keep it balanced. "If I'm drinking wine in the evening, I avoid fruit and fruit juice during the day," she added. So, what's so good about water? Well, what not to love really! Considering that our bodies are made up of over

60% water, we often forget that we need this natural wonder substance to keep us alive and functioning. Here's the thing though: as incredible as our bodies are, it cannot produce all the water that it requires on its own. According to dietician Clare Evangelista, losing just 2% of our water weight due to dehydration can have a significant effect on our physical and mental acuity. That includes water lost through sweating, urinating and even breathing.

"This can affect our response times and muddle our thinking," says Evangelista. "Not drinking enough water can lead to a range of other health issues too – from kidney stones, saggy skin and urinary tract infections to headaches, poor dental health, and hunger pangs."

Need further motivation to get your daily eight glasses in? Let's consider the benefits:

- There's the weight loss element and it's super easy to achieve. "Water contains no calories, so it's very effective if you want to reduce your energy intake and it's a better choice than soft drinks or even a pure fruit juice," according to Barbara Eden of the National Heart Foundation of Australia. "Fruit juice does contain calories and if you are going to drink it, mix it half-half with soda or mineral water to reduce the calorie content." And although we don't advise any sort of quick-fix weight loss programs, filling up on water can go a long way in curbing your appetite. Try sipping on water before sitting down to a meal to satiate your appetite sometime before the food arrives. A study in the United States found that those who consumed two glasses of H20 prior to eating ate far fewer calories at mealtime - up to 90 calories less. This is backed up by Virginia Tech's Dr. Brenda Davy. "Over the course of 12 weeks, dieters who drank water before meals, three times per day, lost about five pounds [2.2 kilograms] more than dieters who did not increase their water intake," she said.

- Worried about your blood sugar levels? Drink water. A study in France surveyed the effects of water of those who consumed four or more daily glasses of water. Compared to users who drank under two glasses per day, the four-a-day group was 21% less likely to contract high blood sugar. And it makes sense too. Dehydration results in a drop in blood volume in the body which, in turn, pushes up the quantity of other elements within the blood like potassium, sodium, and sugar. "Potassium helps control our heart rhythm," says Evangelista. "So, if potassium levels are too high due to dehydration, that can cause heart palpitations."

- If you're feeling tired and fatigued all the time, a lack of water might be to blame. This is especially true in warmer climates when we don't realize just how hard the body needs to work to regulate our core temperature. Once your body goes over the 38-degree mark, feelings of fatigue, lethargy, and nausea are the first symptoms of dehydration. "Water is the best way to replace the fluid we lose.

For any vigorous activity of less than an hour you don't need to drink anything but water," says Eden.

So how do the Parisian It girls get their H20 fix? For Estée Lauder's go-to makeup artist Violette, it's all about herbal water cocktails. Speaking to *Vogue Paris*, she explained: "I never drink tea or coffee, but I like thyme, cranberry and blueberry infusions that help to fight wrinkles."

That said though, heed this advice from Parisian model Cindy Bruna. With typical French insouciance, she told *Coveteur*: "My best advice is not to get too caught up in all this stuff. Eat if you want to eat. Exercise, but in a way that's balanced. Don't find a routine that's difficult; find a routine that's cool. And, remember: water's good but wine is better."

FOLLOW STRICT MEAL TIMES

This one is not rocket science. Eat three regular meals every day and give your body time to digest the nutrients you're feeding it. It makes sense, *non*?

"The French don't eat between meals or on the run and they have distinct meal times," according to nutritionist Dr. Rosemary Stanton. "They have quite small servings and they only eat one rich meal a day. So, if they have a main lunch, they will just have a salad and yogurt in the evening."

"I don't usually snack," agrees Christian Dior publicist Fanny Bourdette-Donon, speaking to *Elle*. "If I can't have a proper meal, I would have a smoothie or fruits to help me wait until I can have a proper meal." If you're persistently eating all the time, you're also constantly thinking about food. This ends up removing the anticipation and pleasure of eating at mealtimes. French children are taught this from a very young age.

In fact, just by looking at the French school dining system, the rest of us can learn a lot about basic nutrition. Consider this: at your ordinary, run-of-the-mill *crèche*, children as young as three years old are served four-course meals akin to the ones you'd expect at a *bistro* (in ceramic cutlery and using "adult" silver cutlery, no less). The meals are typically made up of a salad as a starter, followed by the main course, a selection of cheeses or yogurt and lastly, dessert (mainly made up of fruit pieces).

The principle is that they don't have to finish absolutely everything on their plates, but they have to at least taste everything. "The French believe—and have done scientific research—to prove you can teach your kids to eat just like you teach them to read." So says the author of *French Kids Eat Everything*, Karen Le Billon.

Hey, there's even a government restriction in France that restricts the amount of ketchup that schools are allowed to serve to children on a weekly basis. Other strictly followed guidelines: in the space of one month, only three desserts and four mains are allowed to have a high-fat content of over 15%; fried food can be served a mere four times every four weeks and water is the only beverage to be offered. Cafeteria (or *cantine*) menus are formulated two months prior and sent to a registered nutritionist so that any dietary changes can be made well in advance.

Parents are then encouraged to follow the same philosophy of introducing their children to a wide variety of foods at home. Discovering new tastes and textures are seen as an adventure. Ultimately, the aim is to cultivate an appreciation of foods in all shapes and forms. This is why you won't find children-specific foods in France. Forget chicken nuggets and potato faces. Kids genuinely eat whatever the adults do.

This early education in fine dining results in a healthy, balanced approach to food later in life. Essentially what they are doing is training their bodies into set patterns: when to expect food.

When describing the biggest differences she has noticed between the dietary habits of American and French women, Bourdette-Donon knows her stuff. She explained to *Elle* magazine: "The first thing that comes to my mind is that we don't really eat any type of fried food. We also eat way more portions! We would rather eat many small dishes than a big plate of something. Something really French too is that we can't really eat if we are not seated and have a little time to eat. We can't eat while walking like New Yorkers can, for example. "

There have been conflicting messages over the years with regards to the number of daily meals required to stay healthy. Some proclaim the benefit of five smaller meals spaced throughout the day at set intervals. Others recommend the standard three meals. While each person's metabolism is different, and you are encouraged to follow your own body's signals, consider the scientific evidence. A study by the University of Newcastle found that whether dieters ate three meals per day or six meals, it made zero difference to the amount of weight that they lost.

MAKE AN OCCASION OUT OF IT

Eating in France is a social activity," says Leeds University lecturer Dr. Andrew Hill. There's even a designated term in French to describe the link between food and companionship: *la commensalité* which translates into "being in the company of someone around the table". In fact, the topic of conversation will quite often revolve around the food being eaten. *Ça a quel goût?* (What does it taste like?) *Quel est cet ingrédient?* (What is that ingredient?) *Comment était-il préparé?* (How was it prepared?)

These are not uncommon topics of conversation during a meal and heightens the gastronomic experience, making one really focus on the quality of the food. Children, in particular, enjoy this pastime; a practice that continues long into adulthood.

Just walk past any street-side bistro or terraced brasserie in Paris and you're bound to find clusters of diners animatedly discussing their food. Whether they're dipping crusts of baguette into a frothy bouillabaisse or swirling around an espresso, it's about the *joie* of food.

"There are several but small courses, with plenty of time between courses for the physiological feedback to kick in," adds Dr. Hill. Yes, each portion may be smaller in size but there is variety meaning your taste buds don't ever get bored.

The same applies to snacking throughout the day; a practice frowned upon in France. There are meal times for a reason. Your body needs the time to anticipate and prepare for a meal. Plus, the expectation of a quality meal means that you won't want to ruin your appetite.

Another major no-no: eating in front of the TV. This is simply not done and thought to be crude and uncultured. Speaking of bad manners, here's one to remember lest you want to invoke the wrath of your French hosts. Don't place any type of bread (baguette, brioche etc) on a table upside down. This is thought to bring famine upon your house! This superstition apparently stems back all the way to the time when the town executioner could grab items from shops without paying using only the one hand. Bakers would leave loaves out for them faced upside down.

EAT LIKE A FRENCH WOMAN

"In French, we have a quote that sums up well what a perfect day of eating looks like for me: 'Eat like a queen in the morning, a princess for lunch and a poor girl at night,' says Fanny Bourdette-Donon, bona-fide Frenchwoman and the international publicist for Christian Dior, speaking to *Elle* magazine. That said though, the main mealtime of the day is lunch – this is when you'll have your heaviest proteins and fats. Dinner is kept light. Think salads, soups or a light pasta, followed by yogurt or a piece of fruit.

Author of *French Women Don't Get Fat*, Mireille Guiliano is a firm advocate of this philosophy: "I rely on a few basic rules of thumb: I've said it before, every meal must have the "holy trinity" of carbs, protein, and fat. I also believe lunch should end with a little something sweet (usually fruit, but sometimes a small square of dark chocolate— you can make that call). And, as with every meal, there should always, always, always be pleasure involved."

stuck on a protein to use, think chicken, fish, a ..u-boiled egg, a few ounces of cheese or yogurt. When it comes to carbs, there is bread, of course, but don't rule out some of last night's rice or even a leek and potato soup that you've made over the weekend.

So, what exactly does a French woman eat? These are some of the typical healthy options to be found in the Gallic state, as described by Guilliano. Unless specifically stated, all meals listed serve 4 portions.

Breakfast

Guilliano divulged her typical five-minute breakfast to *Elle* magazine which she adapted from her grandmother's own wonder *petit déjeuner*. What makes it so extraordinary? Combining fiber-rich flaxseed oil, lemon juice, and acacia honey, her crunchy tart creation has everything you need to detox and stimulate your intestine for the day ahead. Keen to give it a go? Take notes:

What you'll need:

- ½ cup of low-fat yogurt
- 1 teaspoon of flaxseed oil
- 1 teaspoon of acacia honey
- 2 tablespoons of raw oatmeal
- 2 teaspoons of walnuts
- The juice of one lemon

Start by pouring the flaxseed oil and lemon juice into the yogurt. Next, drizzle the acacia honey into this mixture. In a separate bowl, mash up the walnuts and oatmeal with a pestle. Mix everything together *et voilà* – a hearty breakfast alternative that will satisfy your carb and sugar cravings. This combination is the perfect size for a single service. For two people, simply double all ingredients. *Parfait!*

Magical Leek Soup

The author counts this as her "magical" recipe and for good reason. She gleaned it from a doctor (who she refers to as Dr. Miracle) who helped her lose a considerable amount of weight when she began her own weight loss journey.

So why leeks exactly? In her own words: "Leeks are a mild diuretic, and 48 hours or so of leek soup would provide immediate results to jump-start the recasting. For me, it was the start of a lifelong commitment to wellness as well as the beginning of my appreciation, my love, of leeks."

What you'll need:

- 2 pounds of leeks (this number depends on your needs, of course. Generally, though, 3 medium-sized leeks are equal to 1 pound. For this recipe, 2 pounds should give you a hearty dose to eat immediately and store away for later).

- A large pot

- Water to cover the leeks

Start by cutting off the leaves (the green bit) as well as the roots at the end. It's the white part you want to cook with. (Don't get rid of the green leaves though - these can be used to make a healthy soup stock later). Then comes the cleaning. Slice the stalk lengthwise, about four-fifths of the way down ending just before the white portion. The vegetable should fan out, revealing the inside. Dip it into a bowl of cold water, making sure to remove any bits of soil in and around the vegetable.

Once they're cleaned, place the leeks in your pot, covering them with water. Leaving the pot uncovered, allow the water to boil for up to 30 minutes. Drain the water and serve the leeks drizzled with extra virgin olive oil as well as lemon juice. Chopped parsley plus salt and pepper can be added to taste.

Gingered Chicken soup

If you're looking for something a little heartier, Guilliano suggests a Gingered Chicken soup, ideal for days when you need a little energetic pick-me-up.

What you'll need:

- 2 pounds of chicken, leg and wing portions
- ½ cup of rice wine
- 8 cups of water
- Fresh sliced ginger to taste

Place the chicken pieces in a large pot and pour over the water, ginger and rice wine. Bring the mixture to a boil before turning the heat down to low. Allow the broth to simmer slowly, leaving the pot uncovered, for an hour and 15 minutes, remembering to stir every once in a while. Strain the soup through a sieve and remove the chicken pieces and ginger. Share the soup between the soup bowls and, just before serving, add the chicken to each bowl and serve.

Spaghetti Alle Vongole

Yes, a plate of carbs is allowed too. Remember Audrey Hepburn's love of pasta? We just know she'd love this seafood-inspired dish!

What you'll need:

- 2 cups of dry spaghetti (that's 500 grams or 1 pound)
- 2 cups of clams
- 3 to 4 cloves of fresh garlic
- 1/2 cup of white wine
- Extra virgin olive oil
- Fresh parsley
- Salt and pepper to season

Start off by cleaning the clams of any dirt while the pasta boils over high heat. In a separate large pot, combine the garlic, parsley and white wine. Toss in the clams. After a few minutes, the shells will have broken open. Remove the clams from the mixture and place aside. Strain the juice left over through a sieve to get rid of any remaining sand and debris. Separate the clams from their shells and add them to a separate saucepan along with the wine mixture. Cover the pan and, over medium heat, allowing it to simmer slowly.

In another saucepan, fry off the second garlic clove in olive oil until brown. At this point, place your cooked pasta into individual bowls, adding the wine and clam mixture. Drizzle your olive oil and garlic mix over this. Season with salt and pepper before finally garnishing with more parsley.

Cucumber Salad with Goat's Cheese

In France, the salad is typically served after the main course and is seen as a palate cleanser to round off the meal before dessert.

What you'll need:

- 2 cucumbers
- 1 clove of finely crushed garlic
- 2 tablespoons of olive oil
- 1 teaspoon of honey
- 1 teaspoon of mustard
- 1 tablespoon of balsamic vinegar
- 1 cup of crumbed goat's cheese
- 1 tablespoon of fresh dill
- 2 teaspoons of sliced almonds
- Salt and freshly ground pepper to taste

Begin by rinsing the cucumbers before slicing them into rounds or even smaller portions if you so desire. In a separate bowl, blend together the olive oil, vinegar, honey, garlic and mustard to make a dressing. Place the cucumber rounds in your individual bowls and sprinkle over the goat's cheese into each bowl. Drizzle the salad dressing over the mixture and season with almonds, salt and pepper and dill.

Chocolate Mousse with Mandarins

Finally, we come to the sweet stuff. This chocolate recipe ticks all the chocolate boxes with an added kick of zesty orange!

What you'll need:

- 100 grams of dark chocolate (60%)
- 2 eggs
- 1 tablespoon of espresso or equally strong coffee
- 2 mandarins
- 1 teaspoon of sugar

Create a bain-marie by melting the chocolate over medium heat in a glass bowl over a pot of simmering water. Once melted, take the chocolate off the heat and add the coffee. Separate the egg yolks and blend them ever so gently into the chocolate, taking care to add them in slowly and one at a time. The egg whites meanwhile need to be beaten until stiff peaks form. Fold the egg whites carefully into the chocolate mix until altogether blended in. Place the mixture in the fridge to chill overnight. At this point, peel the two mandarins, removing the skin and seeds. Place them in a bowl and sprinkle lightly with sugar. Allow those to chill similarly overnight. The following day, they will both be ready to serve: the mousse firm and the mandarins sweet and syrupy.

Blueberry Baby Smoothie

Packed with antioxidants, this pretty purple concoction is great for warm, balmy days but equally as wholesome and nourishing over the cooler, more chilly months.

What you'll need:

- 1 cup of frozen blueberries
- 1 tablespoon of honey
- 1 tablespoon of lemon juice
- 1½ cups of full-fat or 2% milk
- A pinch of ground cardamom

The best part about smoothies? They require minimal effort! Simply blend all the ingredients in a blender and garnish with cardamom right before serving. Perfect!

SMALL DIETARY CHANGES THAT CAN HAVE HUGE RESULTS

- Switch to dark chocolate. Unlike milk chocolate, the darker variety is packed with health benefits as well as considerably fewer calories than its milkier counterpart.

- Drink black coffee. Take your morning brew *sans* the milk and cut out up to 200 calories. That said though, aim for the bare minimum. "Try to limit other tea or coffee to no more than two servings a day, as the caffeine can make you hungry, especially on certain days of the month," says Mireille Guiliano. "It also dehydrates you, and the water in highly caffeinated beverages does not meet the requirement of drinking lots of plain water."

- Start your day with a glass of water, come what may. "When starting her day, a French woman would no more neglect to have her glass of water than to dab a little perfume or eau de toilette on her neck," says Guiliano.

- Instead of limiting yourself to one weekly shopping trip to buy groceries, make a daily habit of it. First, you'll be paying attention to planning that day's meal meaning fresh produce and seasonal unprocessed food. In addition, think of the exercise - traversing up and down the grocery aisles, carrying your parcels to and from the store and unpacking them again. We know, it might sound like a schlep now but for Frenchwomen, it's a way of life.

- We know we've just told you to swap out the milk in your coffee. But not all dairy is bad. Get your fix by consuming a daily dose of cheese. Fun fact: according to the French Committee for Health Education, a tiny amount of cheese is enough to trigger the body's production of cholecystokinin, a hormone which signals to the brain that your stomach is full.

- Change up your lunch menu. You know where cravings come from? A deficiency in one nutrient or food group. This comes from eating the same foods over and over again and skimping out on necessary vitamins and minerals. Experts recommend eating a minimum of 30 varieties of food every week to ingest all the essential nutrients the body requires. If you are eating the same sandwich filling day in and day out... guess what? Your body will feel unsatisfied and drive you to consume more and more until that nutrient is found. Prioritize eating a vegetable-rich lunch every day and feel the difference.

- Toast your bread, especially in the morning. This makes the fiber more digestible plus you won't be wasting any no-longer-fresh slices.

- Speaking of toast, choose organic butter over processed margarine. Your body needs more natural, less processed. Remember that.

- Now-legendary author of the tongue-in-cheek *French Women Don't Get Fat* Mireille Guiliano opts for what she calls "face-friendly" food: "Oysters, honey, and mushrooms (possibly with a glass of bubbly) help put off those dreaded facelifts." Her other favorites: blueberries, yogurt, bread, green vegetables, chocolate and, of course, wine. For anti-aging benefits, she has a foolproof recipe: "beet millefeuille with ricotta and honey". For dessert? "Chocolate soufflés with piment d'espelette."

- If you must snack between meals, have a small tub of yogurt. It will satiate your hunger without compromising your appetite for the main meal to come. Did you know that, of all the nations in Europe, French women consume the most yogurt- a rough estimate of over 48 pounds per year!

- Make your own salad dressing. Never go with ready-made store-bought dressings. "There is no such thing as a good bottled salad dressing," agrees Guiliano. "For salads, I firmly believe the best dressing is a top-quality olive oil and vinegar (1 tablespoon vinegar for 3 tablespoons olive oil, an amount for 2 cups salad). If you need 'spice' in your salad, add a bit of mustard to the dressing, and, of course, always plenty of fresh herbs. "

- Don't overlook a good nutritional supplement. Of course, the best source of nutrients is always fresh produce, but an additional dietary add-on can't hurt either. If you find yourself stressed and frazzled most of the time, a supplement of magnesium might just help you as it did model Camille Rowe. "I definitely noticed a change when I started taking magnesium," she told Into the Gloss. "I get stressed out and crave chocolate all the time, and it's very good about curbing my sweet cravings. And it helps me sleep better."

- Don't fear wine. Enjoy it! And don't bother with so-called dietary pairings either. "If you prefer red wine with fish, go for it. If you don't like wine, you are missing one of the greatest foods on earth, but so be it" says Guiliano.

FITNESS

It's that paradox again. French women never work out yet, by some miracle, they stay svelte and skinny. Ask them how they keep fit and the answers are as wild as they are inventive.

"A French woman is like a wild horse," Estée Lauder makeup guru Violette told *Vogue* magazine. "She is very rebellious, and she'd rather kill herself than go to the gym!"

Asked about her fitness regime, Lola Rykiel (granddaughter of designer Sonia Rykiel) told *Vogue* of her newly-acquired Manhattan-inspired habit of running along the Luxembourg Gardens. "My family thinks I'm so weird—like I'm a real athlete". So how do her Parisian friends prefer to keep fit? "Going out in clubs, walking around Paris, and chilling at cafés! People aren't obsessed with being healthy, most people just are healthy," she said.

"I can't speak for the entire country of France, but in Paris, we have an hour-long lunch break, we go on long walks, we're less stressed," said Rykiel. "The concern is to be who you are and to enjoy life."

Another lover of life is French-American model Camille Rowe (whose mother just so happened to be a dancer at the Moulin Rouge!). "I love a spontaneous solo dance party. I always have music on at home and I'm always shaking a leg,' she told *W Magazine*. "I do yoga every morning. It's become like a meditation to me. I live on a hike, so I'll go for walks once or twice a day. I love an activity!"

In a nutshell, use your body... even if it's only to find your way to the nearest *fromagerie*. Seriously though, what exercises do they do to stay so darn slim? *Allez!*

IF YOU DO NOTHING ELSE, AT LEAST WALK

French women walk.... a lot. The same way that most other nations enjoy the convenience of driving, the French prefer a simple *d'aller à pied*. "I force myself to walk a lot," style guru Caroline de Maigret told *Vogue*. "For example, if I have an appointment and I go by car, I park 20 minutes [away]. Paris is a city where you can walk a lot. Sometimes I just walk for an hour, if I have time, which is the same hour you would have gone to the gym—my mind is happier that way."

Remember too that it's not all that common for a French person to even own a car. In Paris, even less so. Getting around is a case of relying on public transportation or, as most French women do, walk, cycle or take the metro - all of which require a substantial amount of physical activity.

And don't forget the steps! No, we don't mean the Eiffel Tower's impressive 1 700 steps. Most women in Paris live in apartment buildings, the majority of which have several flights of stairs. Elevators are a rare occurrence - don't forget that France is an old country. We're talking Napoleon old when many of the buildings were originally built.

Imagine living on the 12th floor of an apartment building. That's roughly 14 sets of stairs that need climbing several times each day. That's some serious cardio. Add in grocery shopping bags and you've got strength training thrown in for good measure. So how many calories are we talking? Well, let's put it this way: the American Journal of Health Promotion surveyed a group of men and found that walking up stairs eight times per day burned roughly nine calories per minute. Another way of stating it - the same amount as four days of food each year.

Other nationalities would pay good money in monthly gym fees to get the same sort of daily workout. French people, however, don't even consider it to be exercise. It's an unavoidable part of basic everyday life. Plus, there are further far-reaching results of all that trodding. Constant walking means that they feel the need to drink more water which in turn helps to curb their hunger. Win-win!

They also run... occasionally "I run! You have to force yourself at first, but you get addicted very quickly," says Jeanne Damas, talking to *Vogue*. "I have a trainer who comes to my house twice a week and I run along the Coulée Verte in Paris, or wherever I am on holiday."

Another devotee of the Riverside run is French model Charlotte di Calypso. "In Paris, I live right by the Quai de

Seine, where I do a 30 to 40-minute run and 15 to 20 minutes of stronger cardio (exercises)," she told *WomenFitness.net*. "I also bike a lot to go to my appointments, something that I would never do in New York - I am too scared!"

If a jog still feels too much like hard work, think of it as your daily de-stress – a slice of your day dedicated exclusively to rejuvenating your body and refreshing your mind. Founder of the Caudalie beauty range Mathilde Thomas may be based in New York but makes use of her environment to stay fit.

"I never miss the chance to go jogging in Central Park," she told *Vogue Paris*.

Also living in the Big Apple, French-born model Sigrid Agren never steers too far from her Martinique roots. "I find running being the best way to empty my mind," she told the magazine. "Getting a massage really relaxes me too. I go to this amazing beauty therapist in Chinatown for strong massages. It's not fancy at all, but it's the best I've had, I always leave feeling as if I have a new body. Also, a nice cup of hot tea is a simple yet effective way to take a break and relax. I particularly love maté and chai flavors."

LE YOGA FOR LIFE

Yoga is a firm favorite of French women, and it's not hard to see why. "I do yoga as much as I can - it can be hard with work so sometimes I won't be able to do it for a couple of months," said French actress Clémence Poésy, speaking to British *Vogue*. "I also love swimming but it's a case of finding the right pool to go to regularly. It's hard! I do laps, and I just never get bored - if I try to run I just bore myself, I'd have to listen to music or podcasts."

Mathilde Thomas of Caudalie proclaims the wonders of mindful breathing. "I practice breathing exercises and different yoga postures," she told *Vogue Paris*. I would recommend this to anyone suffering from stress."

So where do the who's who of Paris practice their sun salutations? The trendy Omm Studio is situated not far from the Place de Vosges in the creative Marais district. They're known for their gentle, holistic exercises. Bonus: the owner speaks English... always a plus!

But there's also the come-as-you-are, everyone's welcome yoga variety. Located on the open-plan rooftop of the Saint-Ouen Mob hotel, Axelle Roucou leads her yogis in a series of poses with fun and frivolity. And, how French, there is a roomy terrace downstairs as a reward for all your stretching.

A BICYCLETTE

Is there anything more typically French than riding a bicycle? Think back to Yves Montand delightfully crooning *"Quand on partait de bon matin... Quand on partait sur les chemins... A bicyclette..."* to Audrey Hepburn in *Sabrina* and not forgetting Brigitte Bardot's pale blue number in *And God Created Woman*. Or how about the whimsical Miss Dior Cherie advertisement where, directed by Sofia Coppola, the advert's star goes from cheerfully traversing the streets of Paris by bicycle to being swept away by a bouquet of balloons? *Donc très français!*

"In France, we're not the most in love with boot-camp kinds of exercise. But that's why we love bicycles," Marie Laure Fournier told The Cut. "You can see the bicycle trend came from France. My mother is almost 70 years old, and she still bikes! But we don't think of it as exercise. We take the bicycle to go to places."

And it's the perfect fit, we think. After all, the word 'bicycle' itself was first used all the way back in 1847 when a French newspaper struggled to name a never-before-seen two-wheeled mode of transport.

For once, something that both the locals and the tourists can agree on Vélib'. What's that, you ask? With a name roughly translated to mean "bike in freedom", it's just that - the bike rental system that was founded in Paris in 2007. Walk down any street in the bustling capital city and you're bound to spot them. Sleek, matte gray bicycles with reflective yellow discs across the wheels, there are more than 20 000 Vélib' bikes across the city plus 1, 800 rental stations.

There's even an official app that directs you to the nearest bike station as well as the number of bikes available. If you do find yourself renting a Vélib', be sure to invest in a helmet too - if only for your own protection. It's required by law that children under 12 years must wear a helmet but for adults, no such law exists.

So, what about indoor cycling - a fitness trend that's swept across the US? Despite Sonia Rykiel's daughter Lola exclaiming to *Vogue* that "Soul Cycle will never come to Paris" ... alas! There is hope for those who prefer a little more structured exercise. A slew of cycling studios have popped up all over Paris. Unlike the American variety though, at the Paris cult favorite Dynamo, the vibe is decidedly more zen-like. Maybe it's the omnipresent *laissez-faire* attitude that seems to saturate the streets of the city, but the French approach to spinning is akin to yoga. Granted, yoga set to a Beyoncé-driven soundtrack, but still, laidback and peaceful is the point. Oh, and some of the instructors just so happen to be Yves Saint Laurent models to (we're looking at you, Jérémie Laheurte).

Speaking to *The Cut*, Dynamo instructor Clotilde explained the differences she's found in the American versus French approach to fitness. "Yes, I found that Americans can be a little crazy about exercise," she said. "People would be like, I'm going to have kombucha. Meanwhile, I was like, Pff. I'm going to have some wine and maybe some pain au chocolat."

If you can handle something a little more hardcore, there's Let's Ride studio. Much more in line with American standards, this spin spot is set in the edgy 11th arrondissement in the trendy rue d'Oberkampf. The instructor, Steph Nieman, hails from New York so you can be assured an intense 45 minutes of heart-pounding glute, leg and abdominal toning. But, being based in Paris, expect a full *soignée* experience: towels, shoes, and Malin + Goetz skincare products included.

Still not sure? Hunt down the 2013 film *Girl on a Bicycle* for the cutest cycling inspiration, guaranteed.

BOOTCAMP, THE FRENCH WAY

There's a trend catching on in France... first in Paris, but now across the country. It's what's known as bootcamp to the rest of the world, only it's been given a French twist, naturally. Attend a bootcamp anywhere else and you can except the extreme – that is, extreme adrenaline, extreme intensity and, as a result, extreme calorie burning too. These types of grueling outdoor events are generally run by former marines, military cadets, and army sergeants. You get the drill.

And so, when the idea of the bootcamp finally hit the Gallic state, you can rest assured that it was met with some skepticism (and just a hint of eye-rolling too). Paris is, after all, a city renowned for its milder, more holistic approach to exercise - a stroll along the Seine, a light midday yoga class or a scenic bicycle jaunt through the Bois de Boulogne.

Enter Romain Rainaut. In 2014, the Paris native found a unique problem in his hometown: a yearning for fun outdoor exercise that didn't involve expensive fees or stuffy studios. He had just moved back to Paris from London where he had spent 10 years working in finance. Already a fitness devotee himself (having competed in several Ironman competitions) and looking for a change in career, Rainaut and a childhood friend founded Conquer Your Day or CYD.

Advertised solely on Facebook, their first event was a free bootcamp class led by five friends, all of them passionate about fitness. Today the Paris-based initiative has expanded to countless members, with cell groups popping up everywhere from Lille to Marseilles. The classes work like this: those interested in participating connect via a Facebook group. At a pre-arranged time and meeting point, everyone gathers for a 30-minute jog via the city's most picturesque areas. Think Montmartre one day, Pont des Arts the next.

Thereafter comes 25 minutes of specific targeted exercises followed by stretching and a cooling down session. Don't expect professional personal trainers though. The classes are led by *ambassadeurs* - motivated, enthusiastic yet still everyday people. Best of all, it's free. And, because it's Paris, the day is polished off with an after-sweat drink.

BALLERINA GIRL

And then there's ballet. Honestly, could any Parisian workout be more French? This one deserves a try if only for the opulent, authentically French surroundings. BarreShape ballet is held in the hallowed halls of the Éléphant Paname, a lavish mansion from the belle époque days that looks straight out of a French film. The workout itself is an elegant 60-minute mix of ballet with yoga and cardio.

The actual ballerinas of the Paris Opéra are known to visit the popular Studio Kinétique which offers more strenuous multi-faceted full-body workouts such as shiatsu, Pilates, and Gyrokinesis, among others. But this is more than just a gym. Owned by Moraima Gaetmank, a New York expat, and former dancer, and her French artist husband, the studio includes several wellness experts - from a massage therapist to a naturopath - for an all-consuming health experience.

WATER BABY

One active area that the French have wholeheartedly embraced is Aqua Biking. Think of it like spinning on a stationary bicycle except the bicycle is underwater. Originally introduced by Italians as a form of physical therapy, it's the French who have really made the movement (excuse the pun) grow. It only makes sense, right? In a country so well known for its bicycle-peddling antics, it stands to reason that an underwater variety would catch on too.

Too weird for you? Get this: a cardio class can burn in the region of 800 classes per session. Consider all the full-body benefits of cycling: an equal blend of strength and cardio training. The difference with aqua biking though is that there is zero pressure on your joints whatsoever, not to mention the outer thrashing of the water around your legs. You may feel a little silly doing it, but your waistline and your joints will thank you.

FIT NOT FAT

We'd be remiss to discuss fit French adults without paying attention to the way that French children are raised. And it all starts at school. The average school day in France is divided up in such a way that there are three recess times throughout each day: a 15-minute recess in the morning, one long 60-minute break after their lunch and another 15-minute break later in the afternoon. Coupled with that, children typically walk or ride their bicycles to and from school daily.

Then there are the mums. Not to stereotype too greatly, but in other parts of the world, your typical mum will do the school run in her matching gym clothes (whether on her way to the actual gym or not). Not so in France. Remember, there is no real gym culture to speak of. Yes, the athleisure trend may have arrived in the *Ville Lumière*, slouchy dressing-down certainly hasn't. Don't expect to find yoga pants anywhere besides a yoga studio. Gym clothes are for the gym, nowhere else. There are chic everyday clothes and then there are exercise clothes.

"In Paris, wearing leggings during the day is not chic," style blogger Kenza Sadoun-el Glaoui told *Who What Wear*. "If you compare the cities of Paris and Los Angeles, for example, this type of clothing doesn't have much success here. If you see a woman in sweatpants and a sweatshirt in Paris, it shows that she either didn't want to make any effort or on the contrary, that she has a very distinctive style and she owns it. Here in France, we tend to only wear a few activewear pieces at a time—not a sporty total look."

A woman may arrive at a workout class in her Isabel Marant slingbacks but will quickly change into her practical lightweight Nike trainers. The style rules remain the same - understated to a fault. French women are not ones to go out of their way for anything unnatural and affected. Getting fully dolled up to exercise seems exactly that.

Similarly, if you do find yourself in an organized fitness class, you won't find carefully constructed exercise ensembles. No, it's a lot more casual and laidback than that. A boyfriend's oversized T-shirt over basic leggings, or last year's unworn running shorts and half-marathon T-shirt will do just fine. The same goes for trying to one-up your fellow exercisers. A fitness class is about relaxing and getting in touch with your own body, not competing over who can do the best downward dog. Nobody cares whether you have six-pack abs or not. To be honest, the women in a French Pilates class are most likely thinking about which bar will pour them that after-class *apéritif*.

"I do Pilates when I'm in Paris, but being on stage every night is exhausting," Jane Birkin, the legendary doyenne of the French Girl mystique, told the Daily Mail. I'm always running, always late, so that keeps the weight off. If I have time, I do sit-ups, or I do front crawl on the carpet. I can't swim in water - I don't know how - so I do it on dry land. I have to be careful not to get a paunch - I'm so skinny that if I put any weight anywhere, it'd be there, and I don't like a bulge. I wouldn't mind if it went on my bosom, but it doesn't."

There is also a clever service in Paris called So Much More. Although it was started in Germany, the concept has well and truly taken flight in Paris. Essentially, a membership to So Much More or Urban Sports Club is like an address book consisting of over 240 fitness clubs across the city. Staring at €59 per month, you get to choose between 40 different clubs and disciplines at your leisure. Maybe a spot of boxing on Monday? Or how about some lively Zumba on a Saturday morning? One subscription means you'll never be bored in a repetitive workout regime again. And for an always-on-the-move Parisian woman, what could be better?

SMALL WAYS TO INCORPORATE MORE EXERCISE INTO YOUR EVERYDAY LIFE

- You've heard it before and we'll say it again: take the stairs! It might be the easiest way to incorporate a bit of cardio into your day. There is almost always a flight of stairs not too far from an elevator if you look well enough. If given the chance, always take the stairs.

- In a similar vein, if you simply must drive your car, try to park as far away from the entrance as possible. We've all seen those people who drive up and down in parking lots looking for a bay close to the entrance. Don't be that person. Fight the norm and consciously park your car at the edge of the lot... but only if it's safe to do so, of course!

- And once you do find that parking, make sure that your walk to your destination is a brisk, meaningful one. Push your shoulders back, tighten your core and take long, purposeful strides. You'll get in a mini-workout without even really trying.

- Make fitness a priority. Seriously - you could stretch out on the sofa and lament your flabby belly, or you can take little measures to try and fight it. And they needn't be major life changes either. Doing squats while watching the news, or lunges as you do the vacuuming... every little bit helps.

- Here's one that would make grandma proud: start gardening! Yep, you read that right. There's a reason that the previous generation lived to be old and gray - they burned off their calories in the garden! Did you know that the simple task of pulling out weeds can burn up to 200 calories per hour? Impressive, huh?

- Sleep is good, yes. But resist the temptation to sleep in over the weekends and get out in the fresh air. When last have you gone walking around your neighborhood? A favorite pastime of Parisians is simply exploring their streets and suburbs on foot. So, what if you don't live next to the Jardin des Tuileries? Make the best of what you've got!

WELLNESS

Ah wellness: that ubiquitous term that has become a central part of our everyday lexicon. In France, wellbeing is referred to as your *bien-être*, literally meaning "to be good". Unlike in many parts of the world, this idea of conscious and cultivated healthy living is nothing new in France. In fact, a 2013 survey of the OECD countries (a group of 35 developed countries with high-income economies) was conducted by the Centre for Economic and Policy Research. What this research found was that France trumps all other countries when it comes to annual paid vacation days.

On the lowest end of the scale came Japan and Canada who, over a period of one year, offered its workers 10 days of paid leave (although the latter enjoyed an additional nine days of nationwide paid holidays). Straddling the halfway line came countries like Switzerland, the Netherlands, and Germany where workers were given 20 days annually as paid vacation. Then there's France with an unmatched 30 days of annual paid leave (that's an entire month!), seconded only by the United Kingdom with a yearly vacation tally of 28 days.

So where does the United States fall? Surprisingly, of all the countries measured, the US was the only industrialized nation without any sort of legislation on the amount of paid vacation that employers are obligated to provide. Granted, most US employees are given holidays according to their work contract and compensation package; the yearly number averaging at 15 days.

So, do the French know something that the rest of us don't? We think so. In her book *What French Women Know*, American author Debra Ollivier spent 10 years living in France and turned her findings into a book. "They [French women] don't do all the self-fixing that Americans do; they just move on. It's very powerful... Here in the U.S., you must be 'fabulous at 40,''fit at 50,' etc., etc., and it's so stressful. France is a grown-up culture. They like being grown up."

MIND OVER MATTER

Ah, stress - the cause of so many diseases and ailments in the body. Have you ever considered the effect that worry over calories can have on your overall health? Think about a typical meal in your everyday life. Let's say you're preparing an average dinner, either for yourself or for your family. What would your standard thought process be? Perhaps you're thinking about the number of calories you're likely to consume in one sitting? Or maybe you're catering to a houseful of picky eaters – one doesn't like the taste of tomatoes; another can't stand the texture of mushrooms. Perhaps you're simply worried you won't have enough time to prepare a full meal after a long day at work.

Consider this same daily dose of anxiety over the span of a week, a month, even an entire lifetime. Stress of any kind has been well-documented to lead to lifestyle diseases - heart conditions, digestive problems and depression, to name just a few.

Now let's envisage the exact opposite. Imagine planning mealtimes with a sense of anticipation and excitement. It could all be as simple as changing the way you approach mealtimes, whether that's in the preparation or in the eating. Calm down. Take a moment to breathe. It's only food - meant to be one of life's most enduring pleasures. Change the way you think about food and you may just find a newfound joy you had never known before.

THE HERBAL REMEDY

There's a ritual practiced in France that dates as far back Marie Antoinette in the 1700s. No, not eating cake (although a slice of *gateau* is always a welcome addition).

It's called *tisane* and it's like herbal tea. Only... it's not. Unlike other teas which are produced from the *Camellia sinensis* plant, tisane is essentially an infusion of ν parts of plants. And practically every part of plants is used – *tisane* varieties include leaf, root, bark, flower, spice, and fruit. There are even moss-based tisanes... Kombucha *tisane*, anyone?

You can stock up on your desired blend at any French homeopathic pharmacy or *pharmacie homéopathique*, of which there are practically the same number as normal pharmacies. Then there's also the stand-alone *herboristerie* or herbal store where all things natural and herbal are stocked.

Keen to score some *tisane* health benefits? Look out for these herbs:

- For digestive problems, stomach cramps and bloating, try star anise. Place four whole cloves of star anise in a teacup and pour freshly boiled water over it. Cover the cup with a plate, letting the herbs seep for about 10 minutes. Lift out the star anise and enjoy. This works particularly well after a large, heavy meal.

- Is a urinary tract infection getting you down? Find relief in a *tisane* of dried nettle leaves. Blended with boiled water for 10 minutes, this mixture also soothes cystitis.

- To de-stress and relax after a taxing day, a cup of infused boiling water and one tablespoon of culinary lavender will do wonders.

- Then there's the wonderful lime tree. The plant's wild yellow flowers are known to help everything from a fever to reducing anxiety. Let half a tablespoon infuse in a cup of boiling water for 10 minutes before draining and drinking.

STEAM IT OUT

France has a large Turkish community and as a result, hammans have become an essential part of the French woman's relaxation routine. There's the *très* fancy hamman at Le Royal Monceau as well as the more affordable La Grande Mosquée de Paris. Sessions at a typical hamman in France will usually include a full package experience: an intensive sweat session in the steam room, an exfoliating *gommage* or body scrub followed by a full massage, typically half an hour long. Be prepared though - the French hamman massages the entire body (breasts included).

THE POWER OF OHMMMM

Meditation has received a bad rep. The image we've seen portrayed all too often in the media is that of kale-crunching, hippie-esque millennials dilly-dallying in zen-like yoga studios. All that meditation really is, is a focus or mindful focused breathing.

Maybe you've tried quiet meditation and found that it's in fact not for you. A wellness trend that's growing in France is known as Sophrology. It's a meditation-based practice favored by businessmen and models alike, such as Victoria's Secret model Cindy Bruna.

Speaking to *Coveteur*, she explained: "It's like meditation—exercises I do at the gym where I listen to [my trainer]'s voice and do mental work that takes away my stress, gets rid of bad moods and builds my confidence. For example, I'll lie on the floor after a workout, and [he] will tell me to imagine my stress is a cloud—a cloud that's just floating, floating away. Or he'll have me imagine a blue point and focus on that. This type of exercise is very popular in France."

MASSAGE DOES THE BODY GOOD

"I love a good massage," says Garance Doré, talking to *Vogue Paris*. "In an ideal world, I'd have one at least once a week. Not only does it relax me, but it's also a moment of intense creativity for me - I always walk out with about 3,000 new ideas, it's better than daydreaming."

French women are very much about massage - each and every type. And whenever a new one is introduced as the latest must-try innovation, you can be sure that everyone worth their salt will be signed up to try it out. "We are very much completely obsessed with weight!" said beauty publicist Marie-Laure Fournier in an honest chat with *The Cut*. "We will do everything we can to eliminate the first appearance of anything resembling fat or cellulite. But one of the big secrets of the French is lymphatic drainage massage with thoracic therapy."

She added that growing up in France, massage was the biggest insider's secret among the older generation. "I remember when I was a young girl: One of my girlfriends (who was the daughter of a big socialite in France), her mom was in her 40s and had never had an inch of cellulite. She revealed to me that her mom's secret was lymphatic drainage once or twice a week. I did it with her one week — three times. And I actually lost one size."

Keen to give it a go? It's far easier than exercise and much more effective too. "If you have heavy legs or blood-circulation problems, you need to do it," she said. Beware though - it's not for the faint-hearted. "It can hurt like hell," warned Fournier. "It moves your entire body. When I was smoking, I wanted to throw up after I did it. It's moving the toxins out of the body, which is a big shock. Now, I don't smoke so it's easier. But it makes you very tired at the end. The lymphatic system is the toilet system of the body."

STRESS LESS

We get it – this one is easier said than done. You know what, though? Even French women are prone to bouts of worry and angst. The trick is in how they cope with it. The first step is recognizing your stress triggers and then dealing with them timeously. Find those hobbies and pastimes that ease your mind and make you happiest. Prioritize them and set aside time to practice these hobbies regularly. For Parisian makeup artist Violette, that diversion is sketching. "Drawing is a favorite pastime of mine, so I always carry a sketchbook with me," she told *Vogue Paris*. "If I don't have my Sennelier pencils [on] hand, I will sketch using lipsticks and eyeshadows."

"Never let stress eat away at you, or let yourself be brought down by negative people," says photographer Sonia Sieff. But maybe it's Victoria's Secret model, 21-year-old Parisian Cindy Bruna who describes it best. "That's a mantra I apply to all aspects of my life: beauty, fitness, cooking, anything. Keep it simple; keep it cool." *Parfait*!

VANITY IS A POWERFUL TOOL

'Never underestimate the power of a black lace garter belt,' says Anne Barone in her book *Chic and Slim: How Those French Women Eat all that Rich Food and Still Stay Slim*. "[It's] a constant reminder to make choices that pay off in slimness," she says. Funnily enough, she may have a point.

Consider this: there are nearly as many lingerie stores in France as there are bakeries. Names like Princesse Tam Tam, Simone Perele, Etam and Chantal Thomass are some of the highest selling clothing brands in the country.

It's not unusual for women to spend €100 (or more!) on a delicate slip of silk underwear. In fact, it's estimated that the average French woman spends 17% of her clothing budget on lacy underthings. What has this got to do with diet, health, and wellness?

Staying slim and looking their best is a natural way of life for French women, and what better motivation than glamorous lacy lingerie.

"Forget diets,' says Barone. "They are no fun and don't work. What I learned from French women is that ultimately staying slim is not about counting calories or fat grams. It is not about exercise exhaustion. It is really about personal style."

Then there is the frank, open nature of the French that is simply not the norm in other cultures. Never ones to beat around the bush, French friends will do you the favor of letting you know that you look like you've gained weight. A second helping at dinner? Expect the *garçon* to raise his eyebrows at you. It is for your own good, after all.

THE FINE ART OF AGING GRACEFULLY, THE FRENCH WAY

"Aging is a rather American fear—a young country afraid to get old. Here, buildings are old and forever beautiful." This is according to Alice Litscher of the Paris' Institut Français de la Mode where she serves as a professor in fashion communication. "Historically, women's appearances reflected the social status and well being of their home. To this day, if a woman looks chic and sexy, it probably means her husband does well and [that she] is having lots of sex."

This idea is echoed by one of the editors at *Vanity Fair* France, Laurence Vely. Speaking to *Elle* magazine, she explained that, in France, there is no one specific way to be beautiful. "Quirkiness and charm are more valued than a static idea of perfection. In the United States, beauty is almost mathematical and can only be achieved in your 20s." Quite the opposite is true in France. "Once you hit 40, you finally know yourself and what suits you. [You] have real confidence," she says.

Then again it could all come down to perception. French women simply accept that aging is inevitable. Instead of fighting tooth and nail to change what they were born with, they grow into themselves and celebrate this uniqueness. Where does this self-assured sense of identity come from? Simple - they're raised with it.

You've heard the preconception that French women are haughty, stuck-up and arrogant? It's not by accident. When they're young, French girls are taught to be individuals – self-assured and unlike everyone else. They are encouraged to question societal norms and think for themselves, regardless of whether it's popular or not. In fact, no French word even exists for "popular". So, if it seems like a French woman doesn't care about what you think of her, guess what – she probably doesn't.

Let's compare this mindset to just about every other culture. Popularity and the need to be liked by everyone is considered a societal norm, particularly among young girls. As children, they're raised to be "good girls". Opinions are fine if they follow the consensus. And so, a natural complex of inferiority and insecurity festers inside throughout adolescence and into older age. No wonder there is such a fascination and near-obsession with staying and looking young. Anything else is unacceptable.

Cross the pond and the difference couldn't be greater or more apparent. There's a respect and reverence for older women in France (and the rest of Western Europe actually) that is simply not evident in the United States. "The difference is the U.S. is a 'youth' culture, France is not," according to *French Women Don't Get Fat* author Mireille Guiliano. "Literally, here you are old after 30 and not in France. There is still respect for women in their 50s," she says. "I feel young in Paris for the obvious reasons. Men still look at women my age and try to flirt, have humor, low-key, but seduction nevertheless. And what woman is not sensitive to it?"

Look at the media in France, for example. While America exalts youth culture, the French prefer the refinement and elegance that comes with age. In 2014, legendary French actress Catherine Deneuve, then 70 years old, fronted a campaign for Louis Vuitton, along with Caroline de Maigret, aged 39. It makes sense when you think about. The target market for this luxury brand is typically older, more established women able to afford the brand's exclusive apparel.

On describing the unyielding allure of Deneuve, Guiliano was succinct. "When she was young, the picture was different: longer hair, higher heels, often dressed in YSL.

Today, when you see Catherine Deneuve, you still can't help but go 'Wow'. She is a little rounder, but seems to be saying comfortably: 'Who cares? I am the whole package, not an aging neck."

When describing the women that he creates clothing for, fashion designer Guillaume Henry doesn't mince his words. "There's no question of age or body type or even money," he told fashion blogger Garance Doré. Currently the head of design at Nina Ricci, Henry was formerly praised for breathing new life into the legendary vintage House of Carven. He describes his design aesthetic as "fresh" – identifying with the youthful exuberance in all women, regardless of their date of birth. "Fresh is not a question of age. It's a question of identity," he says.

One Last Thing

If you enjoyed this book, you can help me tremendously by leaving a review on Amazon. You have no idea how much this would help.

I also want to give you a chance to win a **$200.00 Amazon Gift card** as a thank-you for reading this book.

All I ask is that you give me some feedback. You can also copy/paste your *Amazon* or *Goodreads review* and this will also count.

Your opinion is super valuable to me. It will only take a minute of your time to let me know what you like and what you didn't like about this book. The hardest part is deciding how to spend the two hundred dollars! Just follow this link.

http://booksfor.review/frenchdiet

[page intentionally left blank]

Made in the USA
Las Vegas, NV
18 March 2022

45890574R00038